CHAIR YOGA

EXERCISES FOR

WEIGHT

Carefully curated and simple simple

Exercises with 28 Days workout plan

to Quickly lose weight

By

Vanessa H. Gourdine

TABLE OF CONTENT

INTRODUCTION

In a world constantly on the move, where time seems to slip through our fingers like sand, Mary found herself caught in the daily hustle. Juggling work, family, and countless responsibilities, she longed for a way to prioritise her well-being without sacrificing precious moments. One day, exhausted and yearning for change, she stumbled upon the transformative world of Chair Yoga for Weight Loss.

As Mary delved into the pages of this empowering guide, she discovered a sanctuary in her hectic life—an oasis where the synergy of mindful movement and ancient yogic wisdom met the convenience of a chair. This isn't just a book; it's a key to unlocking a healthier, more balanced version of yourself. If you've ever felt the weight of the world on your shoulders, wondering how to reclaim your vitality without adding more stress to your plate, you're not alone.

Join Mary and countless others who have embraced the rejuvenating power of Chair Yoga for Weight Loss. This book isn't just about shedding pounds; it's about shedding the burdens that hold you back from living your best life. Let the journey begin, and may the wisdom within these pages not only captivate your attention but also propel you toward a healthier, more vibrant you. Because in the gentle embrace of a chair, you'll find the strength to stand tall, both physically and metaphorically, in the pursuit of your well-being.

SECTION I

CHAPTER 1

BENEFITS OF CHAIR YOGA

Chair yoga is a gentle form of yoga that adapts traditional yoga poses to be performed while sitting on a chair or using a chair for support. This modification makes yoga accessible to people of all ages and fitness levels, offering a wide range of benefits for physical, mental, and emotional well-being.

Accessibility: One of the primary advantages of chair yoga is its accessibility. It allows individuals with mobility issues, seniors, and those with physical limitations to experience the benefits of yoga without the need for getting down on the floor.

Improved Flexibility: Chair yoga promotes flexibility by encouraging gentle stretching and range of motion exercises. It helps to maintain or improve joint flexibility, reducing stiffness and promoting better overall mobility.

Strength Building: Despite the seated position, chair yoga can effectively build strength in various muscle groups. Participants engage in isometric exercises, such as pressing hands together or lifting legs, contributing to increased muscle tone.

Balance Enhancement: Chair yoga incorporates crucial balance exercises, especially for older adults. These exercises help improve stability and reduce the risk of falls, enhancing overall balance and coordination.

Stress alleviation : Chair yoga, much like conventional yoga, centers around breath control and mindfulness, contributing to stress alleviation, mental tranquility, and the cultivation of a heightened sense of overall well-being.

Posture Improvement: Sitting for prolonged periods can lead to poor posture and related issues. Chair yoga encourages awareness of body alignment, helping participants maintain or improve posture, which is essential for spinal health.

Enhanced Circulation: The gentle movements in chair yoga stimulate blood flow, aiding in circulation. This can be particularly beneficial for individuals with sedentary lifestyles or those who experience swelling in the lower extremities.

Emotional Well-being: Chair yoga incorporates meditation and mindfulness practices, fostering emotional well-being. Participants often report reduced anxiety and an improved mood, contributing to a more positive outlook on life.

CHAPTER 2

OVERVIEW OF CHAIR YOGA FOR WEIGHT LOSS

Chair yoga for weight loss is an innovative approach that combines the benefits of traditional yoga with the convenience of seated exercises. While it may not provide the same calorie-burning intensity as some high-impact workouts, it offers a holistic approach to weight management.

Calorie Expenditure: Chair yoga, though low-impact, can contribute to calorie expenditure. The gentle movements and poses engage various muscle groups, burning calories and supporting weight loss goals over time.

Metabolism Boost: Regular practice of chair yoga can help boost metabolism. While it may not result in rapid weight loss, an improved metabolism aids in the efficient utilization of calories and can contribute to a healthier weight.

Mindful Eating: Chair yoga promotes mindfulness and self-awareness, which can extend to eating habits. Being mindful during meals helps individuals make healthier food choices and develop a more positive relationship with food.

Alleviating Stress: The connection between stress and weight gain is well-established. By prioritizing relaxation and stress reduction, chair yoga offers a unique approach to disrupting the pattern of stress-triggered overeating, thereby promoting improved weight control.

Improved Digestion: Certain chair yoga poses involve gentle twists and movements that can aid in digestion. Better digestion can support weight loss efforts by ensuring the body efficiently processes nutrients.

Enhanced Self-Esteem: Chair yoga encourages self-acceptance and body awareness. As individuals develop a positive relationship with their bodies through yoga practice, it can contribute to improved self-esteem, fostering a healthier mindset toward weight management.

Consistency and Sustainability: Chair yoga is accessible to people of all fitness levels and ages, making it a sustainable option for long-term weight management.

Consistency in practice is key, and chair yoga provides a gentle, enjoyable way to stay active regularly.

Chair yoga offers a plethora of benefits, from improved flexibility and strength to stress reduction and emotional well-being. When used as part of a holistic approach, chair yoga can contribute to a healthy lifestyle, including weight management.

CHAPTER 3

GETTING STARTED

Embarking on a chair yoga journey involves more than just physical movements; creating a conducive environment and ensuring correct posture and alignment are vital components. Whether you're a beginner or an experienced practitioner, paying attention to these foundational elements enhances your chair yoga experience.

Setting up a Comfortable Space

Creating a comfortable and inviting space for chair yoga is essential for a positive practice. Consider the following steps to set up an ideal environment:

Choose a Quiet Space: Select a quiet area where you won't be easily distracted. This can be a corner of a room, a peaceful spot in a garden, or any area that allows you to focus without disruptions.

Use a Sturdy Chair: Opt for a stable chair without wheels. Make sure it provides firm support, and the backrest allows for proper alignment during the practice.

Clear the Space: Remove any obstacles or clutter around your chair to ensure a safe and spacious practice area. This helps prevent accidental tripping or knocking into objects during movement.

Enhance Ambiance: Consider adding elements that enhance your experience, such as calming colors, soothing music, or soft lighting. Creating a pleasant atmosphere contributes to a more enjoyable and mindful practice.

Add Props: Depending on your preferences and needs, you can incorporate props like cushions, blankets, or yoga blocks for added comfort and support.

Personal Touch: Customize your space with items that bring you joy or inspiration, such as candles, plants, or meaningful artwork. Personalizing your practice area makes it more inviting and encourages regular use

Proper Posture and Alignment

Maintaining proper posture and alignment is fundamental in chair yoga to ensure a safe and effective practice. Follow these guidelines to establish the correct foundation:

Sit Tall: Begin by sitting at the edge of the chair with your feet flat on the ground. Ground your sit bones, elongate your spine, and engage your core muscles. Sitting tall helps in maintaining a neutral spine.

Align Your Feet: Place your feet hip-width apart, ensuring they are parallel. This provides a stable foundation and promotes balance during various movements.

Relax Your Shoulders: Release tension in your shoulders by gently rolling them back and down. Allow your arms to rest comfortably on your thighs, promoting an open chest and relaxed upper body.

Check Arm and Hand Placement: If your chair has armrests, ensure your arms are comfortably supported without creating tension. Keep your hands relaxed, either on your thighs or in your lap.

Neutral Head Position: Keep your head in a neutral position by aligning your ears with your shoulders. Refrain from tilting your head forward or backward, as this can cause strain on the neck.

Engage Core Muscles: Activate your core muscles by drawing your navel slightly toward your spine. Ensure stability and support for your lower back through this approach. Pay attention to your body's signals and adjust poses accordingly. If a stance becomes uncomfortable or causes pain, modify it to align with your comfort and abilities.

By setting up a comfortable space and prioritizing proper posture and alignment, you lay the foundation for a successful and enjoyable chair yoga practice. These elements not only enhance the physical benefits but also contribute to a holistic sense of well-being and mindfulness during your sessions.

Nutrition Tips

Nutrition plays a crucial role in achieving and maintaining a healthy lifestyle. Whether your goal is weight loss or overall well-being, making mindful food choices is essential. Here, we'll explore healthy eating for weight loss and provide some nutrient-rich snack ideas to support your dietary goals.

Healthy Eating for Weight Loss

Create well-rounded meals with a mix of lean proteins, whole grains, fruits, vegetables, and healthy fats to ensure essential nutrients and control calorie intake. Mind portion sizes by using smaller plates and paying attention to your body's hunger signals. Stay hydrated to avoid mistaking thirst for hunger. Prioritize whole, unprocessed foods for their rich nutrients and fiber. Include lean proteins like poultry, fish, beans, and tofu for muscle maintenance and fullness.

Embrace healthy fats from avocados, nuts, seeds, and olive oil for nutrient absorption. Minimize added sugars and processed foods to avoid excessive calorie intake. Practice mindful eating without distractions to prevent overeating. Plan meals in advance to make nutritious choices easily accessible.

Stick to regular meal times and incorporate healthy snacks for sustained energy levels.

Nutrient-Rich Snack Ideas

Greek Yogurt with Berries: A combination of Greek yogurt and fresh berries provides protein, probiotics, and antioxidants. It's a tasty and satisfying snack.

Vegetable Sticks with Hummus: Pair colorful vegetable sticks (carrots, cucumber, bell peppers) with hummus for a crunchy, nutrient-rich snack that's high in fiber and healthy fats.

Nuts and Dried Fruits: A small handful of mixed nuts (almonds, walnuts, or pistachios) with dried fruits (apricots, raisins) offers a balance of protein, healthy fats, and natural sweetness.

Whole Grain Crackers with Cheese: Choose whole-grain crackers and pair them with a moderate serving of your favorite cheese. This combination provides fiber and protein.

Apple Slices with Nut Butter: Spread almond or peanut butter on apple slices for a delicious and satisfying snack that combines natural sugars with healthy fats.

Hard-Boiled Eggs: Hard-boiled eggs are a convenient source of protein and healthy fats.

Add a dash of salt and pepper to enhance the taste. Create a nutritious and visually appealing smoothie bowl by blending your preferred fruits with Greek yogurt, and garnish it with granola, nuts, and seeds.

Enjoy a sweet and savory protein-rich snack by combining cottage cheese with fresh pineapple chunks for a dose of vitamin C. Steamed edamame makes for a tasty and protein-packed snack; enhance the flavor with a sprinkle of sea salt.

Chia Seed Pudding: Mix chia seeds with almond milk and let it sit until it forms a pudding-like consistency. Top with fresh berries for a nutrient-dense and satisfying treat.

Incorporating these nutrition tips and snack ideas into your daily routine can contribute to a balanced and health-conscious approach to eating, supporting both weight loss and overall well-being. Remember to consult with a healthcare professional or nutritionist for personalized advice based on your individual needs and goals.

SECTION II

CHAPTER 4

CHAIR YOGA POSES

A. Seated Warm-Up Poses

1. Seated Cat-Cow Stretch:
   - Sit with a straight spine, hands on knees.
   - Inhale, arch your back (Cow); exhale, round it (Cat).

- o Repeat for 1-2 minutes, syncing breath with movement.
  - o

2. Seated Side Bend:
   - o Sit tall, raise your arms overhead.
   - o Inhale, lengthen spine; exhale, lean to one side.
   - o Hold for 30 seconds, switch sides.
   - o

3. Seated Spinal Twist:
   - o Sit with spine tall, twist to one side.
   - o Hold the back of the chair with one hand, opposite knee with the other.

o Inhale, lengthen; exhale, twist deeper. Hold for 30 seconds, switch sides.

4. Seated Forward Bend:

   o Sit at the edge of the chair, feet hip-width apart.

   o Inhale, lengthen spine; exhale, hinge at hips and reach forward.

   o Hold for 30 seconds, breathing deeply.

5. Seated Knee to Chest:

   o Sit tall, hug one knee to your chest.

   o Hold for 30 seconds, switch legs.

6. Seated Leg Extension:

- Sit at the edge of the chair, extend one leg straight.
- Flex the foot, reaching towards the toes.
- Hold for 30 seconds, switch legs.

7. Seated High Knees:
   - Sit tall, lift one knee towards the chest.
   - Hold for 15 seconds, switch legs.

8. Seated Marching:
   - Sit with feet flat, lift one knee at a time.
   - Mimic a marching motion for 1-2 minutes.

9. Seated Bicycle Crunches:

- o Sit with hands behind your head, lift knees.
- o Twist torso, bringing one elbow towards the opposite knee.
- o Repeat for 1-2 minutes.

10. Seated Jumping Jacks:

- Sit tall, extend your arms and legs out wide.
- Bring them back to center, repeating for 1-2 minutes.

Remember to maintain slow, controlled movements and focus on your breath. Modify as needed, and consult with a fitness professional or healthcare provider if you have any concerns.

B. Standing Chair Poses

1. Chair Mountain Pose:
   - Stand behind the chair, feet hip-width apart.
   - Inhale, lift arms overhead, palms facing each other.
   - Engage core, hold for 30 seconds.

2. Chair Forward Fold:
   - Stand with feet hip-width, hinge at hips, and reach towards the chair.
   - Let head hang, hold for 30 seconds.

3. Chair Warrior I:
   - Stand facing the chair, step one foot back.

o Bend front knee, lift arms overhead.

o Hold for 30 seconds, switch legs.

4. Chair Warrior II:

o From Warrior I, open hips and arms parallel to the floor.

o Gaze over the front hand, hold for 30 seconds, switch sides.

5. Chair Tree Pose:

o Stand beside the chair, shift weight to one leg.

o Place the sole of the opposite foot on inner thigh or calf.

o Bring hands to heart center, hold for 30 seconds, switch sides.

6. Chair Side Leg Lifts:
    - Hold onto the chair, lift one leg to the side.
    - Lower and lift for 1-2 minutes, switch legs.
7. Chair Knee to Chest:
    - Hold the chair, lift one knee towards the chest.
    - Hold for 30 seconds, switch legs.
8. Chair High Kicks:
    - Stand behind the chair, hold for support.
    - Kick one leg forward, alternating for 1-2 minutes.
9. Chair Standing Twist:
    - Hold the chair with both hands, feet hip-width apart.

- Inhale, lengthen spine; exhale, twist to one side.
- Hold for 30 seconds, switch sides.

10. Chair Calf Raises:

- Stand behind the chair, lift onto toes.
- Lower and lift heels for 1-2 minutes.

Ensure proper alignment in each pose, engage your core, and breathe deeply. Modify as needed, and consult with a fitness professional or healthcare provider if you have any concerns.

C. Core Strengthening Poses

1. Chair Boat Pose:

    o Sit on the edge of the chair, lean back slightly.

    o Lift legs off the ground, balancing on your sitting bones.

    o Extend arms forward, parallel to the ground.

    o Hold for 30 seconds to 1 minute.

2. Chair Plank:

    o Put your hands on the seat and move your feet backward.

    o Maintain a straight line from head to heels, activate your core, and

- o sustain the position for 30 seconds to 1 minute..

3. Chair Knee Tucks:
    - o Sit on the chair, grip the sides for support.
    - o Lift knees towards chest, engaging the core.
    - o Repeat for 1-2 minutes.

4. Chair Leg Lifts:
    - o Sit on the chair with hands on the sides.
    - o Lift one leg straight in front, hold for a few seconds.
    - o Lower and lift for 1-2 minutes, switch legs.

5. Chair Russian Twists:
    - o Sit on the chair, lean back slightly.

- Hold onto the sides, rotate the torso side to side.
- Twist and hold for 1-2 minutes.

6. Chair Side Plank:
   - Position one hand on the chair, raise your hips off the seat.
   - Align your feet or adjust by placing one foot in front.
   - Maintain for 30 seconds to 1 minute, then switch sides.

7. Chair Bicycle Crunches:
   - Sit on the chair, hands behind head.
   - Lift one knee while twisting to bring the opposite elbow towards it.

- o Repeat for 1-2 minutes.

8. Chair Mountain Climbers:
    - o Place hands on the seat, bring knees towards chest.
    - o Alternate legs in a quick, controlled motion for 1-2 minutes.

9. Chair Reverse Crunches:
    - o Sit on the chair, lean back slightly, hands on the sides.
    - o Lift knees towards the chest, engaging lower abs.
    - o Repeat for 1-2 minutes.

10. Chair Hover:
- Sit on the edge of the chair, place hands on the seat.
- Lift hips off the chair, creating a hover.

- Hold for 30 seconds to 1 minute.

Ensure correct posture, take deep breaths, and pay attention to your body. Adjust as necessary, and seek guidance from a fitness expert or healthcare professional if you have any worries.

D. Relaxation and Cool Down Poses

1. Seated Neck Stretch:
   - Sit tall, drop right ear towards right shoulder.
   - Hold for 30 seconds, switch sides.
   - Gently release tension in neck and shoulders.
2. Seated Shoulder Rolls:

- Sit comfortably, roll shoulders in circular motions.
- Inhale as you lift, exhale as you drop.
- Repeat for 1-2 minutes, then reverse.

3. Seated Side Stretch:

- Sit on the edge of the chair, feet flat.
- Inhale, raise arms overhead; exhale, lean to one side.
- Hold for 30 seconds, switch sides.

4. Seated Forward Bend with Chest Opener:

- Sit at the edge of the chair, hinge at hips.

- Interlace fingers behind your back, lift arms and open chest.
- Hold for 30 seconds, breathing deeply.

5. Seated Pigeon Pose:

- Sit tall, cross right ankle over left knee.
- Flex right foot, gently press knee down.
- Hold for 30 seconds, switch sides.

6. Seated Twist with Side Bend:

- Sit with a straight spine, twist to one side.
- Inhale, lengthen spine; exhale, side bend.

- Hold for 30 seconds, switch sides.

7. Seated Butterfly Stretch:
   - Sit tall, bring soles of feet together.
   - Hold feet and let knees drop towards the floor.
   - Gently flap legs for 1-2 minutes.

8. Seated Child's Pose:
   - Kneel on your heels, extend arms forward on the chair.
   - Bend at the waist, bringing chest toward thighs, resting your forehead on the chair seat.
   - Maintain this position for 1-2 minutes.

9. Seated Ankle Rolls:

- Sit tall, lift one foot and roll ankle clockwise.

- Switch direction after 30 seconds, switch legs.

10. Seated Meditation:

- Practice seated meditation by getting into a relaxed position, closing your eyes, and focusing on your breathing.

- Inhale deeply through your nose, exhale through your mouth, and

- repeat for 3-5 minutes to promote a feeling of calmness.

Allow your body to unwind, breathe deeply, and let go of tension during these cool-down poses. Modify as needed, and consult with a fitness professional or healthcare provider if you have any concerns.

E. Balancing Chair Poses

1. Chair Tadasana (Mountain Pose):
   - Stand behind the chair, feet hip-width apart.

- Ground feet, engage thighs, lift arms overhead.
- Hold for 30 seconds, focusing on balance.

2. Chair Tree Pose:

- Stand beside the chair, shift weight to one leg.
- Place the sole of the opposite foot on inner thigh or calf.
- Bring hands to heart center, hold for 30 seconds, switch sides.

3. Chair Warrior III:

- Stand behind the chair, hinge at hips, extend one leg back.
- Keep back straight, arms reaching forward.

- Hold for 30 seconds, switch legs.

4. Chair Dancer Pose:
    - Stand beside the chair, hold onto it with one hand.
    - Lift opposite foot behind, reach opposite arm forward.
    - Hold for 30 seconds, switch sides.

5. Chair Half Moon Pose:
    - Stand beside the chair, extend one leg to the side.
    - Lean towards the chair, reaching the opposite arm overhead.
    - Hold for 30 seconds, switch sides.

6. Chair Eagle Pose:

- Sit on the chair, cross one leg over the other.
- Cross arms at elbows, lift them parallel to the ground.
- Hold for 30 seconds, switch sides.

7. Chair Warrior I with Leg Lift:
   - Stand facing the chair, step one foot back.
   - Lift the back leg, arms reaching overhead.
   - Hold for 30 seconds, switch legs.

8. Chair Side Leg Lifts with Twist:
   - Hold onto the chair, lift one leg to the side.
   - Add a gentle twist towards the lifted leg.

- o Repeat for 1-2 minutes, switch legs.

9. Chair Figure 4 Stretch:

   - o Sit tall, cross right ankle over left knee.
   - o Press knee down gently, keeping back straight.
   - o Hold for 30 seconds, switch legs.

10. Chair Warrior II with Knee Lift:

   - o Stand facing the chair, step one foot back.
   - o Lift the back knee towards the chest.
   - o Hold for 30 seconds, switch legs.

Focus on your breath, fix your gaze for better balance, and be patient with yourself as you explore these balancing chair poses. Modify as needed, and consult with a fitness professional or healthcare provider if you have any concerns.

SECTION III

CHAPTER 5

INTRODUCTION TO SECTION THREE

Integrating Chair Yoga Exercises for Weight Loss into Your Daily Routine

Welcome to the third section of our guide, where we embark on a transformative journey to seamlessly integrate chair yoga exercises for weight loss into your daily routine. This section is thoughtfully curated to provide you with a structured and effective 4-week workout plan, along with tools such as a recording journal and tracker to enhance your experience.

4-WEEK WORKOUT PLAN

Chair Yoga Poses for Weight Loss
Our 4-week workout plan is designed to gradually build strength, flexibility, and mindfulness, contributing to your overall well-being. Each day offers a balance of morning and evening exercises, ensuring a consistent and manageable routine. The exercises are categorized into five sections:

A. Seated Warm-up Poses:

Gentle movements to awaken and prepare your body for the day.

B. Standing Chair Poses:

Incorporating standing elements for added engagement and calorie expenditure.

C. Core Strengthening Poses:

Focusing on your core muscles to enhance stability and promote weight loss.

D. Relaxation and Cool Down Poses:

A crucial part of the routine, helping you unwind and relax after a day's activities.

E. Balancing Chair Poses:

Enhancing coordination and stability, fundamental aspects of a holistic fitness journey.

Daily Exercise Structure

Each day's routine includes two chair yoga exercises—one in the morning and one in the evening. This thoughtful arrangement allows for a balanced distribution of effort throughout the day. Additionally, the categorization of exercises ensures easy tracing and the ability to tailor your workout plan based on your preferences and needs.

Recording Journal and Tracker

To support your journey, we've included a recording journal and tracker. The recording journal provides a space for personal reflections, capturing your experiences, progress, and any insights gained. The tracker serves as a visual guide, helping you monitor your consistency and celebrate achievements.

As you dive into this section, remember that the key to success lies in dedication, mindfulness, and enjoying the journey. Embrace each pose, savor each breath, and let the transformative power of chair yoga guide you towards your weight loss goals. May this 4-week plan be a stepping stone towards a healthier, more vibrant version of yourself. Let's begin this journey together.

Week 1

Foundations of Chair Yoga for Weight Loss

Day 1:

Morning (Seated Warm-up):

Gentle Neck and Shoulder Rolls

Criteria: Slow and controlled movements.

Duration: 2 minutes.

Seated Spinal Twist

Criteria: Gentle twist without strain.

Duration: 1 minute each side.

Evening (Standing Chair Poses):

Chair Squats

Criteria: Controlled descent and ascent.

Repetitions: 10-12 squats.

Warrior I Pose

Criteria: Engage core and stretch arms.

Duration: 30 seconds each side.

Day 2:

Morning (Core Strengthening):

Seated Knee Lifts

Criteria: Lift knees towards chest.

Repetitions: 15-20 lifts.

Boat Pose

Criteria: Lift legs and lean back slightly.

Duration: 20 seconds.

Evening (Relaxation and Cool Down):

Mindful Breathing

Criteria: Deep and rhythmic breaths.

Duration: 5 minutes.

Seated Forward Fold

Criteria: Slowly reach towards toes.

Duration: 1 minute.

Day 3:

Morning (Balancing Chair Poses):

Tree Pose

Criteria: Lift one foot, place sole on inner thigh.

Duration: 30 seconds each side.

Modified Eagle Pose

Criteria: Cross arms and legs.

Duration: 20 seconds each side.

Evening (Rest Day):

Engage in light stretching or mindfulness exercises.

Day 4:

Morning (Full Body Integration):

Sun Salutation Flow

Criteria: Flow through poses with breath.

Duration: 5 minutes.

Child's Pose

Criteria: Relax into the stretch.

Duration: 2 minutes.

Day 5:

- Morning (Balancing Chair Poses):
  - Tree Pose
    - Criteria: Lift one foot, place sole on inner thigh.

- - Duration: 30 seconds each side.
  - Modified Eagle Pose
    - Criteria: Cross arms and legs.
    - Duration: 20 seconds each side.
- Evening (Rest Day):
  - Engage in light stretching or mindfulness exercises.

Day 6:

- Morning (Full Body Integration):
  1. Sun Salutation Flow
     - Criteria: Flow through poses with breath.
     - Duration: 5 minutes.
  2. Child's Pose

- Criteria: Relax into the stretch.
    - Duration: 2 minutes.

Day 7:

- Morning (Seated Warm-up):
    1. Gentle Neck and Shoulder Rolls
        - Criteria: Slow and controlled movements.
        - Duration: 2 minutes.
    2. Seated Spinal Twist
        - Criteria: Gentle twist without strain.
        - Duration: 1 minute each side.
- Evening (Standing Chair Poses):
    1. Chair Squats

- Criteria: Controlled descent and ascent.
      - Repetitions: 10-12 squats.
   2. Warrior I Pose
      - Criteria: Engage core and stretch arms.
      - Duration: 30 seconds each side.

Note:

- The rest day is crucial for recovery, allowing your body to adapt to the new routine.
- As you proceed through Week 1, focus on the quality of each movement.

- Pay attention to your breath and how your body responds to the exercises.

- Feel free to modify any poses based on your comfort level and listen to your body's cues.

Week 2

Building Strength and Flexibility

Day 8:

- Morning (Seated Warm-up):
    1. Seated Shoulder Opener
        - Criteria: Gentle opening of shoulders.
        - Duration: 2 minutes.
    2. Seated Cat-Cow Stretch
        - Criteria: Move spine through flexion and extension.
        - Duration: 1 minute.
- Evening (Standing Chair Poses):
    1. Chair Pose (Utkatasana)

- Criteria: Sit back into an imaginary chair.
      - Duration: 30 seconds.
  2. High Lunge with Chair Support
      - Criteria: Step one foot back, support with chair.
      - Duration: 20 seconds each side.

Day 9:

- Morning (Core Strengthening):
  1. Seated Russian Twists
      - Criteria: Rotate torso from side to side.
      - Repetitions: 15 twists each side.

2. Boat Pose with Leg Extension

- Criteria: Lift legs, extend one at a time.
- Duration: 25 seconds.

- Evening (Relaxation and Cool Down):

1. Seated Meditation

- Criteria: Focus on breath and stillness.
- Duration: 5 minutes.

2. Seated Side Stretch

- Criteria: Reach arms overhead, lean to the side.
- Duration: 1 minute each side.

Day 10:

- Morning (Balancing Chair Poses):
    - Seated Half Moon Pose
        - Criteria: Lift one arm overhead, lean to the side.
        - Duration: 30 seconds each side.
    - Eagle Arms
        - Criteria: Cross arms, palms together.
        - Duration: 20 seconds.
- Evening (Rest Day):
    - Engage in light stretching or mindfulness exercises.

Day 11:

- Morning (Full Body Integration):

1. Chair Sun Salutation

   - Criteria: Adapt sun salutation to chair.
   - Duration: 5 minutes.

2. Seated Forward Bend with Twist

   - Criteria: Twist to one side while folding forward.
   - Duration: 1 minute each side.

Day 12:

- Morning (Full Body Integration):
  - Chair Sun Salutation
    - Criteria: Adapt sun salutation to chair.
    - Duration: 5 minutes.

- Seated Forward Bend with Twist

    - Criteria: Twist to one side while folding forward.

    - Duration: 1 minute each side.

- Evening (Rest Day):

  - Engage in light stretching or mindfulness exercises.

Day 13:

- Morning (Balancing Chair Poses):

  1. Seated Knee to Chest Pose

     - Criteria: Hug knee towards chest.

     - Duration: 1 minute each leg.

2. Seated Tree Pose with Twist

- Criteria: Lift one knee, twist towards it.
- Duration: 20 seconds each side.

- Evening (Full Body Integration):

1. Chair Mountain Pose

- Criteria: Stand tall on the chair, arms overhead.
- Duration: 1 minute.

2. Seated Backbend

- Criteria: Arch back, gaze towards the ceiling.
- Duration: 30 seconds.

Day 14:

- Morning (Seated Warm-up):
    1. Seated Twist with Leg Extension
        - Criteria: Twist while extending one leg.
        - Duration: 2 minutes.
    2. Seated Side Bend
        - Criteria: Reach arm overhead, lean to the side.
        - Duration: 1.5 minutes each side.
- Evening (Standing Chair Poses):
    1. Chair Warrior III Pose
        - Criteria: Extend one leg back, arms forward.
        - Duration: 30 seconds each side.

2. Standing Leg Lifts with Chair Support

   - Criteria: Lift one leg at a time with chair support.
   - Repetitions: 12 lifts each leg.

Note:

- Continue to enjoy the balance of poses and variety in your routine.
- Use the rest day for self-care and reflection on your progress.
- As you move through Week 2, observe any changes in your strength, flexibility, and overall well-being.

- Modify as needed and maintain a mindful approach to each session.

Note:

- Continue to gradually increase the duration or intensity to challenge your body.
- Feel free to customize the plan based on your preferences and comfort level.
- Regularly check-in with your body and adjust the routine as needed.
- Consistency is key to experiencing the benefits of chair yoga for weight loss.

Week 3

Intensifying the Practice

Day 15:

- Morning (Seated Warm-up):
    1. Seated Twist with Leg Extension
        - Criteria: Twist while extending one leg.
        - Duration: 2 minutes.
    2. Seated Side Bend
        - Criteria: Reach arm overhead, lean to the side.
        - Duration: 1.5 minutes each side.
- Evening (Standing Chair Poses):

1. Chair Warrior III Pose

    - Criteria: Extend one leg back, arms forward.

    - Duration: 30 seconds each side.

2. Standing Leg Lifts with Chair Support

    - Criteria: Lift one leg at a time with chair support.

    - Repetitions: 12 lifts each leg.

Day 16:

- Morning (Core Strengthening):

    1. Seated Bicycle Crunches

- Criteria: Bring knee towards opposite elbow.
        - Repetitions: 20 each side.
    2. Plank Pose with Chair Support
        - Criteria: Hold plank position with hands on the chair.
        - Duration: 30 seconds.
- Evening (Relaxation and Cool Down):
    1. Seated Guided Relaxation
        - Criteria: Focus on releasing tension in each body part.
        - Duration: 5 minutes.

2. Legs Up the Chair Pose

- Criteria: Rest legs on the chair, lie on the floor.
- Duration: 2 minutes.

Day 17:

- Morning (Balancing Chair Poses):
  - Seated Knee to Chest Pose
    - Criteria: Hug knee towards chest.
    - Duration: 1 minute each leg.
  - Seated Tree Pose with Twist
    - Criteria: Lift one knee, twist towards it.
    - Duration: 20 seconds each side.

- Evening (Rest Day):
    - Engage in light stretching or mindfulness exercises.

Day 18:

- Morning (Full Body Integration):
    1. Chair Mountain Pose
        - Criteria: Stand tall on the chair, arms overhead.
        - Duration: 1 minute.
    2. Seated Backbend
        - Criteria: Arch back, gaze towards the ceiling.
        - Duration: 30 seconds.

Day 19:

- Morning (Balancing Chair Poses):
  - Seated Knee to Chest Pose
    - Criteria: Hug knee towards chest.
    - Duration: 1 minute each leg.
  - Seated Tree Pose with Twist
    - Criteria: Lift one knee, twist towards it.
    - Duration: 20 seconds each side.
- Evening (Rest Day):
  - Engage in light stretching or mindfulness exercises.

Day 20:

- Morning (Full Body Integration):

1. Chair Mountain Pose

   - Criteria: Stand tall on the chair, arms overhead.
   - Duration: 1 minute.

2. Seated Backbend

   - Criteria: Arch back, gaze towards the ceiling.
   - Duration: 30 seconds.

Day 21:

- Morning (Seated Warm-up):

  1. Seated Twist with Leg Extension

     - Criteria: Twist while extending one leg.
     - Duration: 2 minutes.

2. Seated Side Bend

- Criteria: Reach arm overhead, lean to the side.
- Duration: 1.5 minutes each side.

- Evening (Standing Chair Poses):

1. Chair Warrior III Pose

- Criteria: Extend one leg back, arms forward.
- Duration: 30 seconds each side.

2. Standing Leg Lifts with Chair Support

- Criteria: Lift one leg at a time with chair support.

- ■ Repetitions: 12 lifts each leg.

Note:

- These days continue to emphasize the holistic approach of chair yoga.
- Use the rest day for light activities that promote relaxation.
- As you approach the end of Week 3, acknowledge your progress and commitment.
- Stay present in each pose, and remember to modify based on your individual needs and comfort level.

Note:

- Keep pushing your limits by extending the time and trying different approaches.

- Pay attention to your body and make adjustments accordingly.

- Maintaining consistency and staying mindful are crucial elements for ongoing improvement.

Week 4

Mastery and Continuation

Day 22:

- Morning (Seated Warm-up):
    1. Extended Seated Forward Bend
        - Criteria: Reach arms forward, lengthen the spine.
        - Duration: 2.5 minutes.
    2. Seated Cat-Cow Flow
        - Criteria: Flow through cat-cow movements.
        - Duration: 1.5 minutes.

- Evening (Standing Chair Poses):

    1. Chair Warrior II Pose

        - Criteria: Extend arms, gaze over front hand.

        - Duration: 40 seconds each side.

    2. Standing Side Leg Lifts with Chair Support

        - Criteria: Lift one leg to the side with chair support.

        - Repetitions: 15 lifts each leg.

Day 23:

- Morning (Core Strengthening):

    1. Seated Leg Circles

- Criteria: Circle legs in both directions.
        - Repetitions: 10 circles each direction.
    2. Side Plank with Chair Support
        - Criteria: Lift hip, support with hand on the chair.
        - Duration: 40 seconds each side.
- Evening (Relaxation and Cool Down):
    1. Guided Body Scan Meditation
        - Criteria: Systematically relax each body part.
        - Duration: 6 minutes.

2. Seated Wide-Legged Forward Bend

- ■ Criteria: Fold forward with legs wide apart.
- ■ Duration: 2 minutes.

Day 24:

- Morning (Balancing Chair Poses):
  - Seated Extended Hand-to-Big-Toe Pose
    - ■ Criteria: Extend one leg forward, and reach for the toe.
    - ■ Duration: 45 seconds on each side.
  - Seated Crow Pose

- Criteria: Lean forward, and lift your feet off the ground.
        - Duration: 30 seconds.
- Evening (Rest Day):
    - Engage in light stretching or mindfulness exercises.

Day 25:

- Morning (Full Body Integration):
    1. Chair Dancer Pose
        - Criteria: Hold one foot with the opposite hand.
        - Duration: 1 minute on each side.
    2. Seated Pigeon Pose

- **Criteria:** Cross ankle over the opposite knee, hinge forward.
- **Duration:** 1.5 minutes on each side.

Day 26:

- Morning (Seated Warm-up):
    1. Seated Twist with Leg Extension
        - **Criteria:** Twist while extending one leg.
        - **Duration:** 2 minutes.
    2. Seated Side Bend
        - **Criteria:** Reach arm overhead, lean to the side.

- - Duration: 1.5 minutes each side.
- Evening (Standing Chair Poses):
  1. Chair Warrior III Pose
     - Criteria: Extend one leg back, arms forward.
     - Duration: 30 seconds each side.
  2. Standing Leg Lifts with Chair Support
     - Criteria: Lift one leg at a time with chair support.
     - Repetitions: 12 lifts each leg.

Day 27:

- Morning (Core Strengthening):

1. Seated Bicycle Crunches

    - Criteria: Bring knee towards opposite elbow.

    - Repetitions: 20 each side.

2. Plank Pose with Chair Support

    - Criteria: Hold plank position with hands on the chair.

    - Duration: 30 seconds.

- Evening (Relaxation and Cool Down):

    1. Seated Guided Relaxation

        - Criteria: Focus on releasing tension in each body part.

- Duration: 5 minutes.

2. Legs Up the Chair Pose

- Criteria: Rest legs on the chair, lie on the floor.

- Duration: 2 minutes.

Day 28:

- Morning (Balancing Chair Poses):

1. Seated Knee to Chest Pose

- Criteria: Hug knee towards chest.

- Duration: 1 minute each leg.

2. Seated Tree Pose with Twist

- Criteria: Lift one knee, twist towards it.

- Duration: 20 seconds each side.
- Evening (Full Body Integration):
  1. Chair Sun Salutation
     - Criteria: Adapt sun salutation to chair.
     - Duration: 5 minutes.
  2. Seated Forward Bend with Twist
     - Criteria: Twist to one side while folding forward.
     - Duration: 1 minute each side.

Note:

- Congratulations on completing this 4-week chair yoga journey!

- Feel free to continue incorporating these exercises into your routine.
- Modify and adapt based on your comfort level and preferences.
- Embrace the mindful and holistic approach to well-being.

Final Note:

- Congratulations on reaching the culmination of this 4-week chair yoga journey.
- Feel free to continue exploring and adapting these exercises to your preference.
- Remember, the journey doesn't end here; it's the beginning of a

sustainable and mindful approach
to your well-being.

CHAPTER 6

JOURNAL AND TRACKER USER GUIDE

Welcome to the "Journal and Tracker User Guide" for our Chair Yoga Weight Loss Book. This comprehensive guide spans four weeks and is designed to enhance your chair yoga experience. Inside, you'll find dedicated sections for tracking your workouts and reflecting on your progress.

The exercise tracker provides a structured layout for each day, allowing you to plan your morning and evening sessions. Checkboxes are provided to mark off completed exercises, helping you stay organized and visually track your daily accomplishments.

Following each week's tracker, you'll discover reflection pages. These pages serve as a space for documenting challenges, milestones, motivation, and emotions. Engaging in this reflective dialogue allows you to connect with your past, present, and future self—a testament to your commitment and growth.

Beyond the initial four weeks, extra tracker and reflection pages enable you to continue your chair yoga practice. This journal transcends its pages, symbolising your dedication to fitness and the limitless possibilities that lie ahead. Let it be a source of motivation, inspiring you to maintain consistency and celebrate your achievements throughout your chair yoga journey.

Chapter 7

TRACKER AND JOURNAL

DAYS	EXERCISES	CHECK

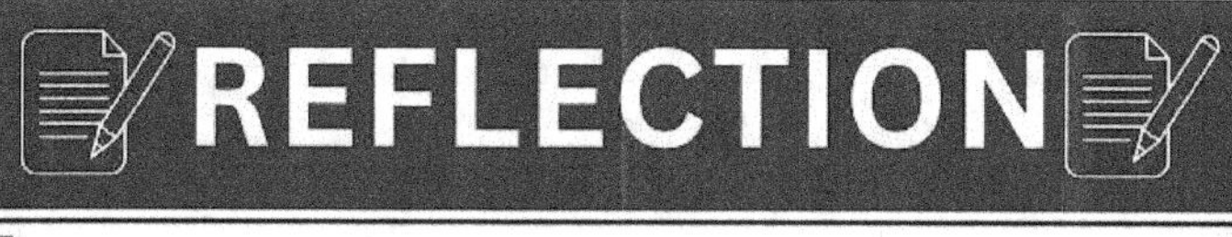

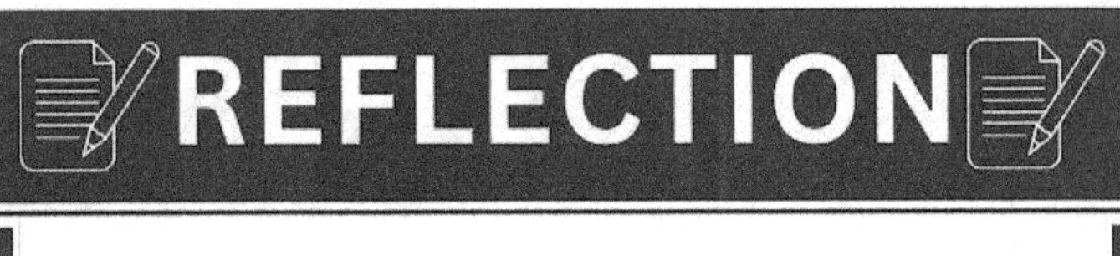
REFLECTION

REFLECTION

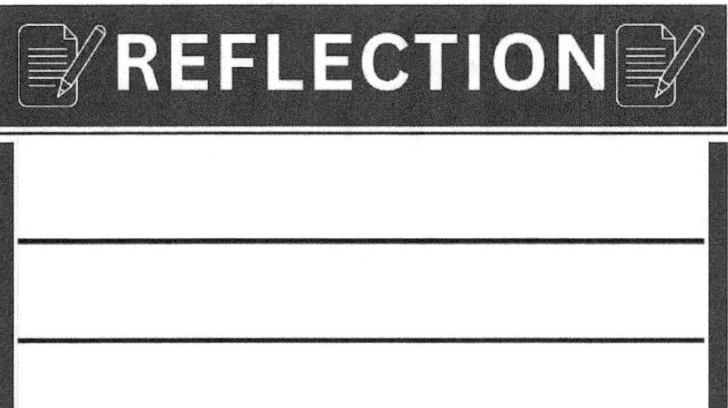

REFLECTION

DAYS	EXERCISES	CHECK

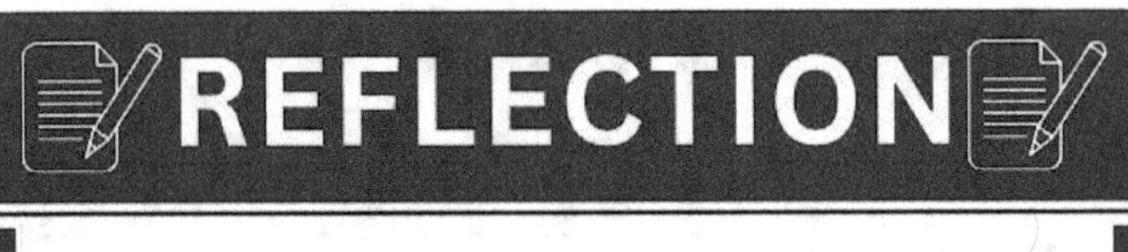

REFLECTION

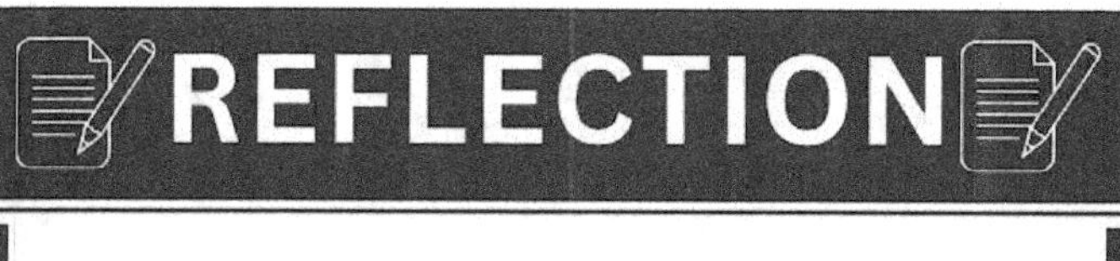
REFLECTION

REFLECTION

REFLECTION

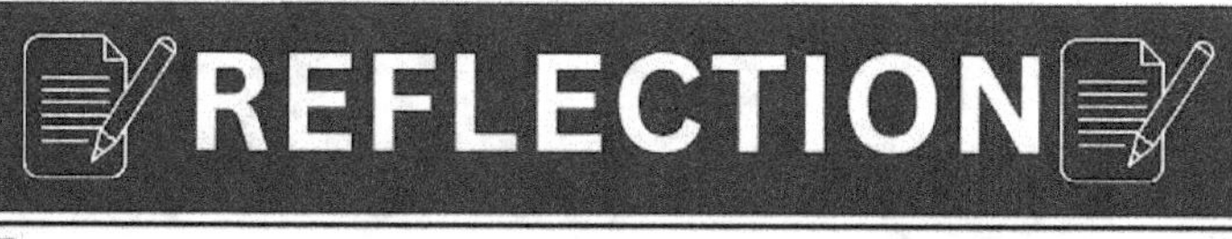

DAYS	EXERCISES	CHECK

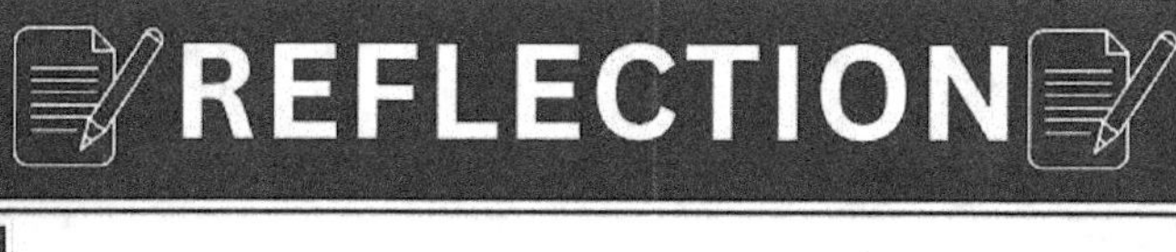

REFLECTION

REFLECTION

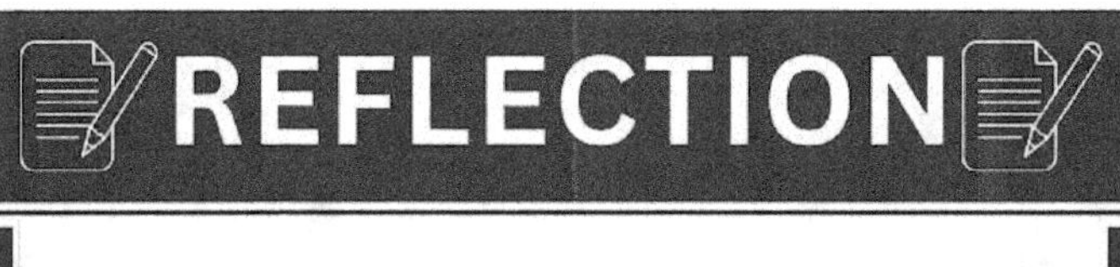

REFLECTION

REFLECTION

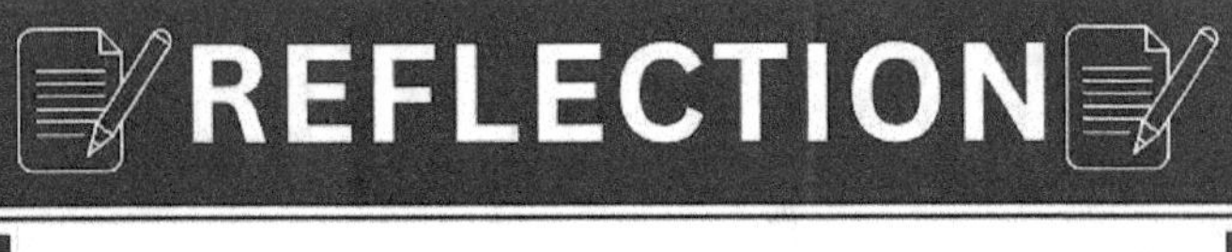

DAYS	EXERCISES	CHECK

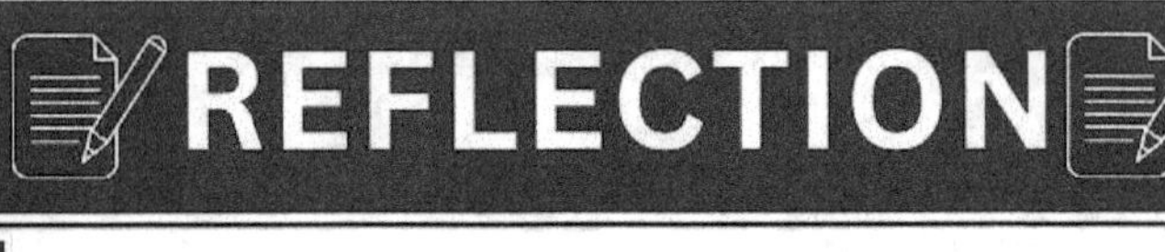

REFLECTION

REFLECTION

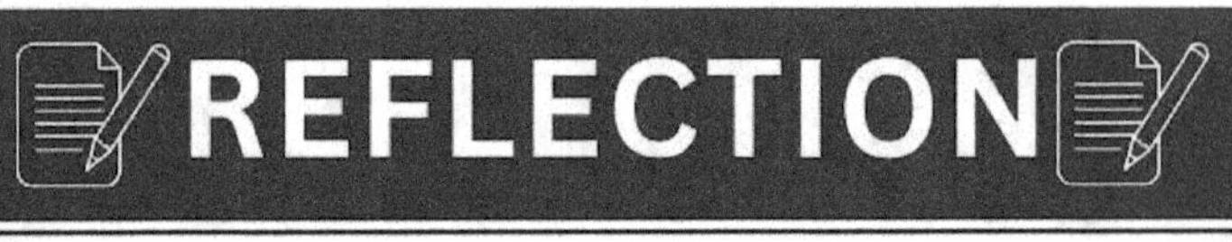

REFLECTION

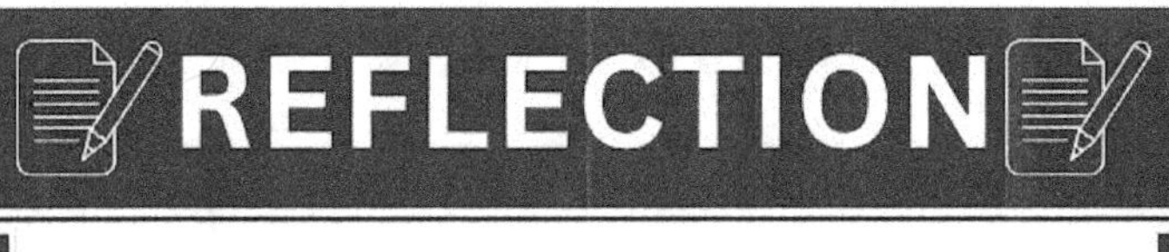

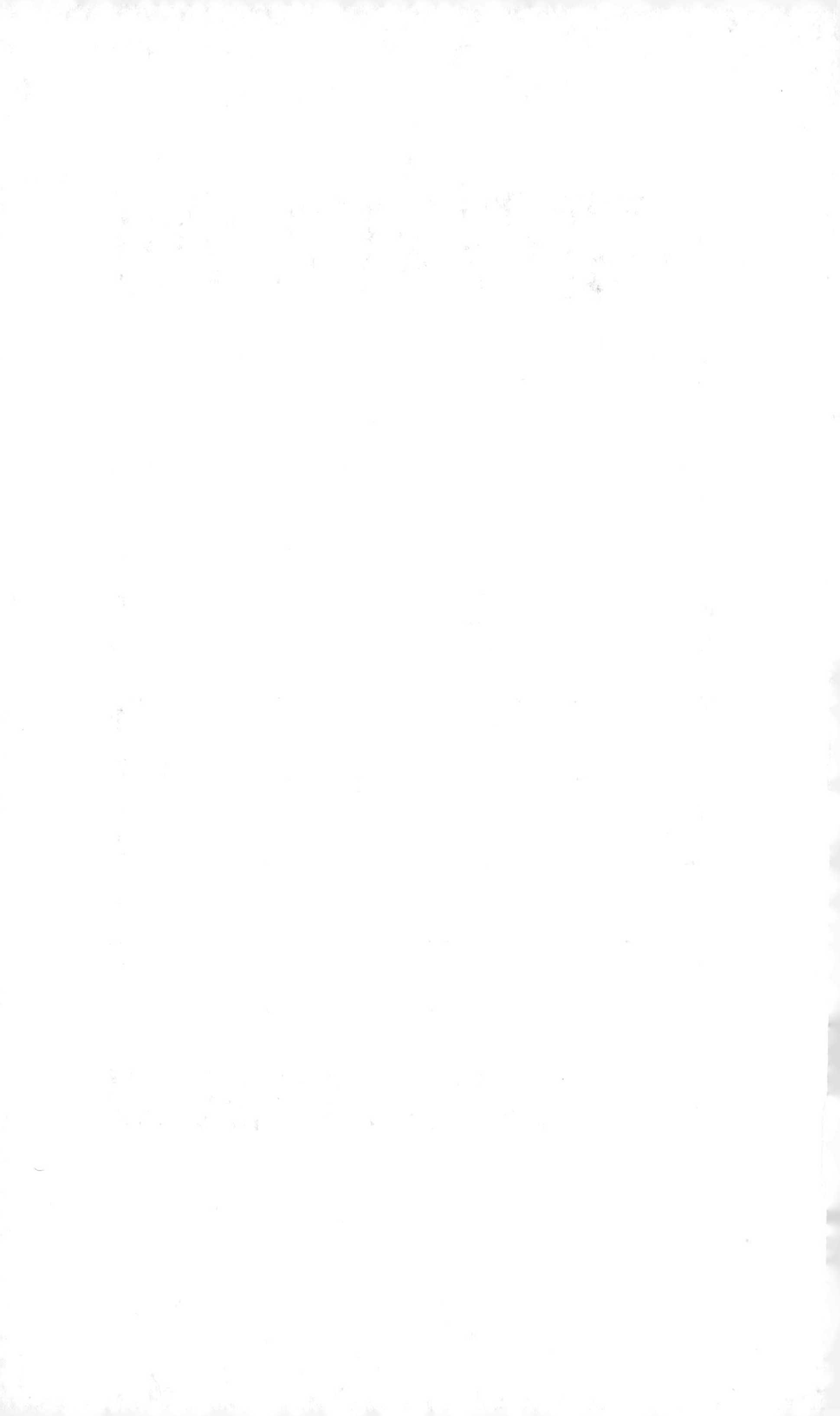